MY TUMMY HAS A HEADACHE

Helping Children Understand Illness

COMPILED BY

Beverley Mathias
and
Desmond Spiers

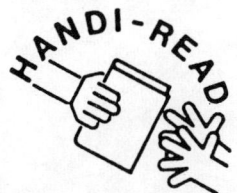

National Library for the Handicapped Child
Reach Resource Centre

Published by the National Library for the Handicapped Child
Reach Resource Centre

This booklet copyright © NLHC 1993

Produced by Signpost Books 1993
Typeset by DP Photosetting, Aylesbury, Bucks
Printed by Risboro Printers Ltd, Princes Risborough, Bucks

ISBN 0 948664 15 0

logo copyright Nederlands Bibliotheek en Lektuur Centrum

No part of this publication may be reproduced, stored in a retrieval system, or transmitted in any form or by any means, electronic, photocopying, recording, or otherwise, without the written permission of the publisher.

Cover illustration from TEDDY BEARS AND THE COLD CURE by permission of Susanna Gretz and A & C Black

The National Library for the Handicapped Child gratefully acknowledges the financial support of
Tixylix Paediatric Medicines

INTRODUCTION

Finding a title for this, the second of our publications, has been quite a challenge, and it is still not exactly right. All children suffer from illness at some point in their lives, whether it be a simple cold or meningitis, a viral infection or tonsillitis, but suffering the illness itself is not the only thing that needed to be included in this particular list.

Children do not only fall ill, they become sufferers, either long or short term, of a variety of conditions that need medical care. Asthma, eczema, epilepsy and glue ear are now common enough in childhood to be included in publications such as this.

Then there are accidents and other reasons for attending hospitals: inoculations, medical and dental checks; visits to the optician, the speech therapist and the many other people who assist in the wellbeing of children. All of these events impinge on the child's health, and could loosely be classed as illness.

Children, especially those under the age of five, are often not very good at explaining why they don't feel well, which means parents and carers have to conduct a 'twenty questions' interrogation. So the title of this handbook reflects the dilemma many adults find themselves in when trying to discover why a child is sick. The all-embracing word 'illness' has been used to cover a multitude of reasons why a child might need medical attention.

This handbook has been compiled because there is now more awareness of the need to explain to children and their parents, the treatment and long-term prognosis for a number of conditions children suffer. For this reason cancer has been included, but terminal illness is not covered. That is included in *A Handbook on Death and Bereavement* published by NLHC in 1992. This new list covers the positive aspects of health care, including hygiene, preventive medical treatment, and general care of sick children. Some titles can be used to discuss certain conditions and aspects of an illness, but this is not their primary use. Books should be available for children to find when they want them, and preferably before the event rather than after it.

Books can be used to overcome or explain a situation, for example, the titles in this collection which cover deafness and the use of hearing aids; or glasses and sight. There are titles which will help to prepare children for a visit to the hospital, either for day surgery or a longer stay. The work of doctors, nurses, therapists is explained in general terms so that the child is prepared for what each person might ask them to do.

In one or two cases, an illness or condition has been included which is not strictly a childhood complaint, such as schizophrenia. This does affect children, but the only title which seems to be available is about a parent. We have included it because it gives a clear and simple explanation of the condition. AIDS is a topic which cannot be ignored, and there are three titles included in this list. One is fiction, the others are factual and designed to be used with groups of children as discussion topics. They are by no means the only information on AIDS available for children. In the list of helpful organisations you will find an address to write to for further information.

Genetic conditions such as Down's Syndrome have been excluded, not because they are unimportant, but because they will probably be included in a more relevant publication.

Difficulties with sight and hearing have been included because they affect so many children. Glue ear is common, and many children need to wear glasses at school. Hearing loss is covered both generally and more specifically under the keyword 'hearing aid'. Because of the confusion which can arise over loss of sight, blindness and the wearing of prescribed glasses, two headings are used – 'sight' and 'glasses'. Blindness is not used as a heading. 'Sight' covers all aspects of sight and vision, including care of the eyes.

Inoculation for childhood complaints has been included, often it can be found within a book covering medical check-up, but vaccination for travel has been excluded, as this is not common to a great number of children.

Hospitals are covered generally rather than by specific departments, although there are biographical studies of some hospital specialists. The need is to allay fear in children and explain what happens when you are admitted to hospital or taken to casualty. For this reason ambulance work has been included as this is often the first contact a child will have with a hospital, and is usually experienced when the child is traumatised.

Where the illness is a side issue to assist the plot of a story, the book has been indexed under the section which covers the greater percentage of the book. So although there is one title which mentions appendicitis, it is included in the books about hospital care. This also applies to other books, especially those covering a number of illnesses or conditions. All books about a topic are listed under the same keyword, which means that picture books, fiction, non fiction and books for adults are all listed together. Some books are listed more than once, where it was thought important to mention more than one aspect. For instance books about hearing aids will also be listed under 'hearing', and books listed under 'inoculation' may also be listed under 'doctor'.

The arrangement is alphabetical by title with an alphabetical author index, an alphabetical keyword index and a listing of useful organisations.

Hopefully, this list will prove useful to teachers and parents, therapists, hospitals, and care workers who are concerned about helping children to understand illness, chronic conditions and just feeling sick.

Some of the titles included here are out of print. It is a fact of life that publishers are no longer able to keep large stocks of titles in print and therefore print runs are often small. Almost every title in this collection should be available through public or school libraries even if it can't be purchased. A number of titles are not currently published in Britain, and it will be noticed that quite a number come from one particular American company, Albert Whitman. Anyone finding difficulty in purchasing these titles should contact the compilers for help.

Although every attempt has been made to find all suitable titles, the compilers would be very pleased to hear of any others which readers think should be included in the next edition.

KEY TO ABBREVIATIONS OF EDITIONS

Hb — hardback
Pb — paperback
Lp — large print
F — Fiction
NF — Non Fiction
Pic — Picture Book

KEY TO AGE INTEREST LEVELS

Ps Preschool
I   Infant
Lp Lower primary
Up Upper primary
S   Secondary
A   Adult reference

1 ACCIDENT
Krailing, Tessa
Davis, Jon
Macmillan, 1989, 0 333 46898 8 Pb
Rocky is fooling around on the swings in the local park when he falls off the swing and knocks himself unconscious. His friend Jamila goes to get help from Fred. While Fred calls the ambulance, Jamila goes and finds Rocky's mum. Rocky is taken in an ambulance to the hospital and Jamila and his mum follow in a police car. Rocky is kept in hospital under observation for a few days to make sure there are no hidden complications.
Lp, Up, F

2 AFRAID TO ASK: A BOOK ABOUT CANCER
Fine, Judy
Kids Can Press, 1984, 0 919964 79 6 Hb
Kids Can Press, 1984, 0 919964 56 7 Pb
In a practical and easily read style, the author sets about explaining what cancer is, and some of the many forms it can take. Using interviews with cancer patients and their families, she asks questions and elicits honest answers. The various treatments are explained and the prognosis of the more common cancers is given. There is a bibliography, but as this is a Canadian title, some of the books mentioned might not be available in the United Kingdom.
A, NF

3 AIDS
Hawkes, Nigel
Franklin Watts, 1987, 0 86313 632 X Pb
This is one of the titles in the Issues series looking at problems which affect children, and offering topics for discussion. Although written some years ago, this still has relevance today as it talks about the issues involved in combatting and preventing the spread of the disease. No moral stance is taken and the effort is made to show all views of the condition, including the ways in which it can be transmitted.
Up, S, A, NF

4 ALEX, THE KID WITH AIDS
Girard, Linda Walvoord
Sims, Blanche
Albert Whitman, 1991, 0 8075 0245 6 Hb
To begin with, Alex feels that because he has AIDS his anti-social behaviour in class can be excused. As the children learn through teachers and the school nurse that playing with Alex won't infect them, they become less lenient towards his teasing. After a particularly cruel taunt, Alex realises that if he wants to be accepted as part of the class he must learn to behave in a more understanding manner towards his friends.
Lp, Up, NF

5 ALL ABOUT ASTHMA
Ostrow, William & Vivian
Albert Whitman, 1989, 0 8075 0276 6 Hb
William Ostrow explains that his asthma started when he was eight years old. He then explains what asthma is, how it affects him and the medicines he takes to make life easier.
Up, S, NF

6 ALLERGIES AND THE HYPERACTIVE CHILD
Rapp, Doris J
Thorsons, 1988, rev ed., 0 7225 1608 8 Pb
There has been much research regarding the interconnections between allergies and hyperactivity. In many cases it has been proved that a child's difficulties are food related, and a period of time without certain known

irritants has resulted in calmer behaviour. In this book the author looks at the research and discusses both sides of the argument regarding hyperactivity and food allergies, plus other controversial issues relating to behaviour. Included are suggestions for diet plans to help parents discover which substances might be affecting their child. The appendices offer ways of ensuring the home environment is free of allergy triggers.
A, NF

7 AMBULANCE CREW
Cooper, Alison & Bentley, Diana
Fairclough, Chris
Wayland, 1990, 1 85210 851 7 Hb
Ron and Sharon work on an ambulance, and are seen getting the vehicle ready for a day's work, checking the equipment and supplies that it carries. They receive a 999 call to collect a pregnant woman whose baby is arriving sooner than expected. After this they go to a garage to treat a workman who was injured when a piece of equipment fell on him. He is given a drip and has a tube inserted in his throat to help him breathe while he is being rushed to hospital.
I, Lp, NF

8 AMBULANCE DRIVER
Wood, Tim
Fairclough, Chris
Franklin Watts, 1989, 0 86313 823 3 Hb
A basic introduction to the work of an ambulance driver, with clear photographs and a short text in large print. Some detailed facts are given at the end of the book and there is a glossary to explain some of the words used.
I, Lp, NF

9 THE AMBULANCE WOMAN
Stewart, Anne
Fairclough, Chris
Hamish Hamilton, 1985, 0 241 11680 5 Hb
Kate is an ambulance woman and for part of the time she is rostered to transport day patients to and from hospital. On these days she works

alone. She checks the equipment before she leaves and keeps a record of her journeys. On other days she works with the emergency ambulance crews. The text and photographs show her and her partner Ian as they respond to two emergency calls.
I, Lp, NF

10   ANN VISITS THE SPEECH THERAPIST
Snell, Nigel
Hamish Hamilton, 1983, *0 241 11029 7* Hb
A very simple and 'comforting story' of a small girl with a speech difficulty. Ann first goes to the doctor, and then to see a speech therapist because Mum is worried about her speech. At the speech clinic Ann begins to learn how to say certain sounds, she practises at home and watches as Mum makes the same sounds for her.
I, Lp, NF

11   ARTHUR'S LOOSE TOOTH
Hoban, Lillian
Heinemann, 1988, *0 434 94402 5* Hb
Arthur and his little sister Violet are being looked after by the baby sitter. Arthur has a loose tooth and can't wait for it to come out so he can get 10p from the tooth fairy, but he is worried in case it falls out without him knowing. He tries to pull it out himself, with a rather painful conclusion.
I, F

12   ARTHUR'S TOOTH
Brown, Marc
Piccadilly Press, 1986, *0 946826 48 X* Hb
Arthur is still the only one in class who has not lost any of his baby teeth and he feels left out. The rest of the class make fun of him, especially Francine. His loose tooth just stays there no matter what he does, but it is Francine who solves the problem in the end.
I, Lp, Pic

13 ASTHMA IN CHILDHOOD
Milner, A D
Nathanson, David
Churchill Livingstone, 1984, 0 443 02652 1 Pb
This is the fifteenth in a series of handbooks dealing with childhood conditions. Asthma is explained in simple terms using both text and diagrams. Some of the more commonly used medications are also discussed. Using a question and answer technique, the author attempts to cover all aspects of this condition, pointing out that of all asthmatic children only 3 per cent will need long term treatment.
A, NF

14 AT THE DOCTOR
Grunsell, Angela
Forsey, Chris
Franklin Watts, 1983, 0 86313 051 8 Hb
A simple story explaining what happens to a child who is ill and has to go to the doctor. The boy in the story has his temperature taken, pulse checked, throat and ears looked at. He is allowed to listen to his own heart with the doctor's stethoscope. Finally he has an X-ray which shows he has a chest infection. He has to stay in bed for a few days and take some pills.
Ps, I, Lp, NF

15 BEN'S BRAND-NEW GLASSES
Dinan, Carolyn
Faber, 1987, 0 571 14567 1 Hb
Ben can't see very well. Although the optician helps him to select a nice frame, he won't wear his new glasses. Despite trying hard to lose them in a variety of ways, the glasses always seem to find their way home bringing with them some new friends. Eventually, when his teacher appears in new glasses, Ben decides to give them a try.
I, Lp, Up, Pic

16   BIG JIM, LITTLE JIM
Cunliffe, John
Beach, Michael
Andre Deutsch, 1990, 0 223 98552 2 Hb
Grandfather and grandson — Big Jim and Little Jim — are the best of friends and do many things together. They both become ill and need to go into hospital, but refuse to go. It is up to Gran to come up with a plan that will get both the Jims into hospital. After they come out they tell their friends that hospital wasn't bad and they are glad to feel so much better.
I, Lp, Pic

17   BRINKWORTH BEAR GOES TO THE DENTIST
West, Annie
Blackie, 1992, 0 216 93258 0 Hb
Blackie, 1992, 0 216 93257 2 Pb
Brinkworth Bear has a good time when he goes to the dentist and even learns a rhyme for brushing his teeth. Simple pictures and rhyming text make this book fun. The print is 10mm in height with no more than twenty words to the page.
Ps, I, Pic

18   BRINKWORTH BEAR GOES TO THE DOCTOR
West, Annie
Blackie, 1992, 0 216 93256 4 Hb
Blackie, 1992, 0 216 93255 6 Pb
With no more than fifteen words to a page, this rhyming story with print 10mm in height is a good book to use with a young child. Bertie has an earache and mum takes him to see the doctor. He has his throat, ears and chest checked. He's given a medicine to drink morning, noon and night.
Ps, I, Pic

19   A BUTTON IN HER EAR
Litchfield, Ada B
Mill, Eleanor
Albert Whitman, 1976, 0 8075 0987 6 Hb
Angela's parents suspect she has a hearing loss because her responses to their speech make no sense. She is taken to the doctor for an examination and is referred to an audiologist for some tests. The

audiologist confirms that she has a hearing loss and that she will require a hearing aid. On the first day she wears it at school teacher asks her to explain to the other children what it does and how it works, so they will have a better understanding of hearing loss. The teacher says that there is no difference between wearing glasses or a hearing aid.
Lp, Up, NF

20 BUTTONS THE DOG WHO WAS MORE THAN A FRIEND
Yeatman, Linda
Casson, Hugh
Piccadilly Press, 1985, 0 946826 95 1 Hb
Colt Books, 1990, 0 905899 02 4 Pb
Philip is deaf, does not speak and is lonely. When he is given a puppy he starts to take an interest in life. Sadly the puppy goes missing and Philip is devastated. Unknown to Philip, Buttons is found and taken to a dogs' home where he is selected for training as a Hearing Dog for the Deaf. His training regime is explained and is interesting. Eventually Buttons is ready to be given to a new owner and this turns out to be Philip.
Lp, Up, F

21 A CANE IN HER HAND
Litchfield, Ada B
Mill, Eleanor
Albert Whitman, 1977, 0 8075 1056 4 Hb
Valerie has always worn glasses to help her to see, but one day she finds that her sight is regressing. The doctor confirms her fears and she realises that life will have to change. Her teacher introduces her to a peripetatic teacher, who helps Valerie with mobility training and using a long cane. Despite her increasing lack of usable vision, Valerie remains in mainstream education with a classroom assistant.
Up, NF

22 THE CHECKUP
Oxenbury, Helen
Walker Books, 1983, 0 7445 0038 9 Hb
Walker Books, 1988, 0 7445 0986 6 Pb
A little boy does not want to visit the doctor for a checkup. None of the

other patients waiting for the doctor wants to speak to him and he has to be dragged into the surgery. He still won't co-operate and the situation ends with the doctor needing some sticking plaster.
Ps, I, Pic

23   A CHECKUP WITH THE DOCTOR
Smith, Katherine, A
Magic Beans, 1989, 0 947212 29 9 Pb (Large Format)
Magic Beans, 1989, 0 947212 30 2 Pb
The book explains what happens when you go for a checkup and illustrates some of the instruments the doctor might use when examining you — tongue depressor, thermometer, sphygmomanometer etc.
I, Lp, NF

24   CHILDREN WITH CANCER: A MODEL OF CARE
Carleton, Don
CLIC Publications, 1990, 0 9515876 0 9 Pb
This title is more an outline of the standard of care preferred for children with cancer and their families than an explanation of the condition. CLIC works for the families, offering accommodation and support, while also encouraging the changes in hospital routine which allow a child a more relaxed environment in which to be treated, and hopefully recover.
A, NF

25   CHILDREN'S HAEMOPHILIA BOOK
Bruna, Dick
Concept Partnership, 1990, 2nd ed., No ISBN, Pb
Written with the help of a group of mothers who have haemophiliac sons. The book explains what the condition is and gives some basic guidelines for the parent to give to the child so that he knows what to do if he has an accident. The book will help the child understand that he can do practically all the things his friends can do and that there are no major problems for anyone living with haemophilia.
Ps, I, NF

26 CLAIRE'S GYMNASTIC POODLE
Yeatman, Linda
Owen, Angela
Piccadilly Press, 1990, *185340 045 9* Hb
Claire has an asthma attack for the first time and suddenly her life changes. She is not allowed to do any more gymnastics and Curly her poodle is sent away. However as tests are carried out to find what triggers the asthma attacks, Claire is slowly allowed to restart many activities, but most importantly her dog is returned.
Lp, Up, F

27 CLARE HAS AN EAR INFECTION
Pattison, Andrew
Barrett, Virginia
Hyland House, 1988, *0 947062 32 7* Hb
Clare wakes up one morning with a very sore ear, so mum takes her to see Dr Toby. After looking at her ear, examining her chest and throat, the doctor says she has an ear infection and will have to take some antibiotics to make it better.
I, Lp, NF

28 COOL SIMON
Ure, Jean
Orchard Books, 1990, *1 85213 213 2* Pb
Corgi Books, 1992, *0 552 52707 6* Pb
Simon has a hearing problem. His speech is not always clear, and he sometimes has trouble understanding what the teacher is saying, particularly when the teacher turns his back. This doesn't stop Simon taking part in any antics that are going on.
S, F

29 COPING WITH SKIN AND HAIR PROBLEMS
Leigh, Dr Irene & Wojnarowska, Dr Fenella
Chambers, 1985, *0 550 20506 3* Pb
Skin conditions such as eczema and psoriasis are discussed at length, with basic facts given for a number of common skin problems such as acne. The connection between skin conditions and allergies is discussed and treatments suggested. Also discussed are cosmetic treatments for

dealing with scars, moles and other permanent or temporary skin disorders.
A, NF

30 CROMWELL'S GLASSES
Keller, Holly
Hippo Books, 1987, 0 590 70722 1 Pb
Nobody wants to play with Cromwell, he's clumsy and he gets lost. Because he is a short-sighted rabbit, Cromwell needs glasses, but he isn't quite old enough. Eventually the time is right, his eyes are examined and he is given glasses. Once he can focus and see what is happening, he discovers the joys of playing with his friends.
I, Lp, Pic

31 THE DEAREST BOY IN ALL THE WORLD
Lieshout, Ted van
Puffin, 1993, 0 14 036238 X Pb
Tim is seven and a worrier — how to look after his mother and sister now that his father is dead, how his sister will cope with her asthma. Tim comes up with a plan that solves all his worries — for a while.
Lp, Up, F

32 DENTIST
Wood, Tim
Fairclough, Chris
Franklin Watts, 1988, 0 86313 648 6 Hb
A first introduction to a dentist and the people who help her in the surgery. A look at dental hygiene and a patient having a hole in her tooth repaired. An X-ray machine is also seen in use.
I, Lp, Up, NF

33 DIABETES IN YOUR TEENS
Farquhar, J W
Churchill Livingstone, 1982, 0 443 02220 8 Pb
The teenage years are fraught enough without the diagnosis of a condition which is going to need constant monitoring. This is a positive look at diabetes, the problems and the treatments, but most of all it is a guide for teenagers facing the regime of insulin and diet control. This

advice includes information about sexual activity, pregnancy and family planning.
S, A, NF

34   THE DIABETIC CHILD
Farquhar, J W
Churchill Livingstone, 1981, 0 443 02193 7 Pb
Written basically for the parents of diabetic children, this book describes the stages from diagnosis through initial treatment to self management of the condition. Also included is information about schooling, respite and residential care, food and exercise, and the effect of diabetes on other family members.
A, NF

35   DINOSAURS ALIVE AND WELL: A GUIDE TO GOOD HEALTH
Brown, Laurie Krasny & Marc
Collins, 1991, 0 00 184738 4 Hb
Using dinosaurs, this attractive picture book explains through text and pictures how to keep yourself healthy. It advocates cleanliness, exercise of mind and body, sensible eating habits, and no worrying. Also included is simple first aid, plus tips for dealing with your feelings. The authors make it very clear that some first aid is beyond the capabilities of children and indicate when it is time to call in a grown-up.
Lp, Up, NF

36   DOCTOR TOBY
Pattison, Andrew
Barrett, Virginia
Hyland House, 1988, 0 947062 30 0 Hb
A young boy introduces Dr Toby, his family's doctor, whom he has known since he was a baby. Some of the staff of the medical centre are also mentioned: Barbara the receptionist, and some of the special doctors to whom Dr Toby can send his patients. The boy is very comfortable visiting Dr Toby and wants to know how he too can become a doctor.
I, Lp, NF

37 DON'T CALL ME FATTY
Philips, Barbara
Cogancherry, Helen
Blackwell Raintree, 1991, 0 86256 003 9 Hb
Being overweight at any age is not good for mental or physical health. Rita is plump, and objects to being called 'Fatty', so she accepts the help offered by her parents. As a family they begin to change their diet and to exercise regularly. Rita sometimes succumbs to temptation, but as she recognises her improving skill in the swimming pool she begins to see the value of the changed regime. The school health check confirms her weight loss. An important point is made by the school doctor who makes sure Rita understands that growing children need to eat well and shouldn't lose too much weight.
Lp, Up, NF

38 EPILEPSY: THE DETECTIVE'S STORY
Rogan, Peter
Hollomby, David
Quay Pubs., 1990, 1 85642 008 6 Pb
Debbie has a hidden disability — epilepsy — and wants to find out more about it. With her parents she goes in search of some answers. She finds that many famous people in history have had epilepsy, including Julius Caesar and Napoleon, and that there are different types of epilepsy — Grand Mal, Petit Mal, Temperal Lobe, to name three. She also finds out what an EEG is and how the results are interpreted. Apart from a few activities such as climbing, Debbie can do the same things as her friends. Finally she is given some guidelines to show her friends what they should do if she has a fit while with them.
Lp, Up, NF

39 EPILEPSY EXPLAINED
Laidlaw, Mary V & John
Churchill Livingstone, 1980, 0 443 01962 2 Pb
From diagnosis to management, this book details the stages and answers the most commonly asked questions. There are descriptions of the varying types of epilepsy and the possible side effects of certain drugs. Public awareness is also discussed together with the issue of employment and marriage. The information given is factual and practical.
A, NF

40 EVEN LITTLE KIDS GET DIABETES
Pirner, Connie White
Westcott, Nadine Bernard
Albert Whitman, 1991, 0 8075 2158 2 Hb
A young girl talks about living with diabetes from the age of two. She explains how she has to have a blood sample taken four times a day to check if she has too much sugar or insulin in her blood. At the moment, mummy or daddy give her the insulin injection, but when she is older she will do it herself. She says she is an ordinary child, though she's sometimes cross at not being able to eat sweets and cakes.
I, Lp, NF

41 FLYING DOCTOR
Pepper, Susan
Fairclough, Chris
Franklin Watts, 1985, 0 86313 317 7 Hb
A book about a more unusual side of the medical profession, the Flying Doctor Service, which operates in some of the isolated parts of Australia. We see the planes that are used, the equipment that they carry, and the medical treatment they carry out at patients' homes. Sometimes treatment has to be given in the air on the way to the main base and hospital.
Lp, Up, S, NF

42 FROM ASTHMA TO THALASSAEMIA: MEDICAL CONDITIONS IN CHILDHOOD
Curtis, Sarah (ed.)
British Agencies for Fostering & Adoption, 1987 0 903534 69 X
This is an alphabetically arranged listing of the most common medical conditions found in children, ranging from arthritis and deafness, to schizophrenia and sickle cell disease. For each condition information is given regarding diagnosis and treatment, plus schooling and prognosis. A list of organisations is appended to each entry.
A, NF

43 GEORGE GETS CHICKENPOX
Snell, Nigel
Hamish Hamilton, 1984, 0 241 11298 2 Hb
George is looking forward to going to Bobby's birthday party, but isn't feeling very well so has to go to bed instead. The next morning he wakes up covered in spots and the doctor has to be called. Chickenpox is diagnosed.

Ps, I, NF

44 GERMS MAKE ME SICK
Berger, Melvin
Hafner, Marylin
A&C Black, 1989, 0 7136 309 2 Hb
With a simple straightforward text and plenty of pictures, the authors explain what germs are, where they might be found, and what happens when germs make you sick. No specific illnesses are mentioned, and the text does make it clear that viral infections can't always be cured through the use of medicine. Coughs, colds, 'flu and chickenpox are talked about as being germ-based illnesses. The bulletin board at the end gives handy hints for staying away from germs.

I, Lp, Up, NF

45 GIDEON AHOY!
Mayne, William
Windrush, 1988, 1 85089 967 3 Hb, Lp
Viking, 1987, 0 670 81165 3 Hb
Puffin Plus, 1989, 0 14 032129 2 Pb
Gideon is sixteen and as a result of contracting meningitis at a young age is deaf, intellectually handicapped and without intelligible speech. His family understand the few sounds he does make. A family friend offers Gideon a job working on a canal barge. It takes him a while to get the hang of things and despite a nasty accident, everything is going well until he decides to use his initiative. How his disability affects his family, especially his younger sister, comes across very well in the story.

S, F

46 GLASSES, WHO NEEDS 'EM?
Smith, Lane
Viking, 1991, 0 670 84313 X Hb
An unconventional look at the wearing of spectacles. A boy goes to the

optician to have his sight checked and finds that children are not the only beings who wear glasses. The text layout at times resembles an optician's chart. The list of those who wear glasses becomes more and more surreal as the boy and the optician vie with each other, until eventually the boy is persuaded that glasses will help him see.
Up, Pic

47   GOING INTO HOSPITAL
Althea
Stubbs, Joanna
Dinosaur Publications, 1986, 0 85122 539 X Pb
A simple story explaining what might happen if you have to go into hospital. It explains what a children's ward is like and that sometimes parents can stay the night as well. If no parent accommodation is available they will still be able to visit. A child on a drip, another one having an X-ray, a girl being prepared for an operation to remove her tonsils are all shown in the ward.
Ps, I, NF

48   GOING TO THE DENTIST
Civardi, Anne
Cartwright, Stephen
Usborne, 1992, 0 7460 1516 X Hb
Usborne, 1992, 0 7460 1515 1 Pb
Jake has toothache and his mum takes him and his sister Jessie to the dentist. Jessie has her teeth examined first and there are no problems. When Jake's teeth are examined the dentist finds a small hole, which is why he was in pain. The dentist gives Jake an injection in the gum, drills out the tooth and then fills it. Before the children go home he tells them how to look after their teeth by eating the right food and brushing their teeth regularly.
I, Lp, NF

49   GOING TO THE DENTIST
Petty, Kate
Kopper, Lisa
Franklin Watts, 1988, 0 86313 676 1 Hb
Sam and his sister Jenny are both a little scared to be going to the dentist.

Jenny sits on mum's knee while the dentist looks at her teeth. In the meantime, Sam has discovered that the dentist's chair goes up and he is keen to sit on it so that the dentist can look at his teeth. Sam has a hole in one of his teeth which requires a filling. He also has an X-ray which shows a new tooth ready to come through to replace one of his baby teeth.

I, Lp, NF

50   GOING TO THE DOCTOR
Civardi, Anne
Cartwright, Stephen
Usborne, 1992, 0 7460 1506 2 Hb
Usborne, 1992, 0 7460 1505 4 Pb

Jack has hurt himself and Jenny is not feeling very well so mum makes an appointment at the surgery for that morning. Jack has to have his arm put in a sling and is told to wear it for a few days. Jenny has her throat, ears and chest examined and is told that she has a slight infection and will need to take some medicine. Baby Joey is given his next inoculation.

Ps, I, NF

51   GOING TO THE DOCTOR
Petty, Kate
Kopper, Lisa
Franklin Watts, 1987, 0 86313 583 8 Hb

Dad takes Sam to see the doctor for his regular checkup — height and weight measured, sight tested. He then has to have an inoculation and though he doesn't like injections he is very brave.

Ps, I, NF

52   GOING TO THE HOSPITAL
Civardi, Anne
Cartwright, Stephen
Usborne, 1992, 0 7460 1512 7 Hb
Usborne, 1992, 0 7560 1511 9 Pb

Ben has earache and goes to the doctor. The doctor says he needs to have an operation on his ear so he is taken into hospital. He gets settled into the children's ward with the help of his mum. A nurse then checks his pulse, temperature and blood pressure to make sure they are normal.

Mrs Hart, the surgeon, comes and explains to Ben what will happen during the operation. After the operation he is able to get out of bed and play with the other children.
I, Lp, NF

53 GOODBYE DOESN'T MEAN FOREVER
McDaniel, Lurlene
Bantam Books, 1991, 0 553 40368 0 Pb
Melissa has leukaemia and her best friend Jory is finding it very difficult to accept. We follow Jory fighting her own feelings of confusion over her friend's illness and the fact that Melissa will eventually die. This is a companion volume to 'Too Young To Die'.
S, F

54 HARRY WITH SPOTS ON
Powling, Chris
Anderson, Scoular
Black, 1990, 0 7136 3224 0 Hb
Young Lions, 1991, 0 00 673884 2 Pb
After skilfully organising the school trip to go where he selected — the Adventure Park — Harry develops measles and cannot go. However, his imaginative mum and dad manage to make the school trip day an event nobody will forget.
Lp, F

55 HEALTH AND HYGIENE
Ward, Brian R
Franklin Watts, 1988, 0 86313 666 4 Hb
This title from the Life Guides series discusses some of the common causes of infection including measles, mumps and chickenpox. It also looks at parasitic infections such as round worm, tape worm and head lice. Photographs of children suffering from these conditions are shown. The text is clear and well illustrated with both photographs and drawings. There is a double page spread giving the names and details of a number of common and less common illnesses.
Up, S, NF

56 HEALTH, ILLNESS AND DISABILITY
Azarnoff, Pat
R R Bowker, 1983 *0 8352 1518 0* Hb
In this bibliographic reference book, the author evaluates and describes numerous children's books, both fiction and non-fiction, which deal with illness, health care and disability. Each title included has been selected because of its factual, positive and helpful attitude to the condition under discussion. Subjects covered include hospitalisation, childhood illness, preventive health care and visits to doctors, dentists and therapists. The arrangement is alphabetical by author with both subject and title indexes.
A, NF

57 HEALTHY EYES
Jackman, Wayne
Wayland, 1990, *1 85210 927 0* Hb
A clearly written and illustrated factual book on looking after your eyes and sight. Good colour photographs show children using their eyes, wearing protective goggles, putting in a contact lens and wearing glasses. A small section explains colour blindness, and there is a brief piece about blindness, guide dogs and independence.
Lp, Up, NF

58 HEARING
Jackman, Wayne
Fairclough, Chris
Wayland, 1989, *1 85210 734 0* Hb
One of a series of books looking at the different senses. In *Hearing* different types of sounds are investigated. It includes simple experiments to explore hearing, explains how hearing is tested, how speech is acquired, and the different functions of human ears and animal ears.
Lp, Up, NF

59 HEARING
Pluckrose, Henry
Franklin Watts, 1985, *0 86313 280 4* Hb
Simple text and clear colour photographs help the child to understand

what hearing is, how the ear works, some of the problems that can occur with the ears and the remedies for these.
I, Lp, NF

60 HELP FOR BED WETTING
Meadow, Roy
Churchill Livingstone, 1980, 0 433 02236 4 Pb
A common complaint which is often kept quiet within the family, and sometimes no help is asked for or offered. This slim volume explains the physical reasons why a child or adult might wet the bed on a regular basis, and offers some of the treatments used to control and cure the difficulty. The problem is dealt with sensitively and constructively by the author, who has many years of experience in dealing with the complaint.
A, NF

61 HELP ME, MUMMY, I CAN'T BREATHE
Sutherland, Susan
Souvenir Press, 1987, 0 285 65035 1 Hb
Souvenir Press, 1987, 0 285 65036 X Pb
A mother's story of the development of asthma in her young child, the treatment received, both medical and authoritarian, and the fight for correct diagnosis. Part of this book has been reconstructed from diaries kept by the author and part comprises practical explanations and suggestions for helping with the various problems faced by parents of asthmatic children.
A, NF

62 THE HICCUP CURE
Goldman, Dara
Piccadilly Press, 1989, 1 85340 049 1 Hb
Red Fox, 1991, 0 09 971950 9 Pb
Sam likes to scare everybody, but one scare backfires and he ends up with the hiccups. His friends come up with many cures including drinking water and blowing into a paper bag. Molly solves the problem by scaring Sam, but then *she* starts hiccuping!
Ps, I, Pic

63 HOSPITAL
Colherne, John
Fairclough, Chris
Franklin Watts, 1987, 0 86313 611 7 Hb
An introduction to different hospital departments and the people who work there — nurses, cooks, scientists, doctors, the outpatients department, and the children's ward. The photographs are very clear and the text simple with no more than four lines per page.
I, Lp, NF

64 HOSPITAL
Vaughan, Jenny
Macmillan, 1989, 0 333 45971 7 Hb
Twenty-one chapters which look at all aspects of the work in a hospital. Apart from current practices in the UK, there is an historical survey of illness and examples of medical practice in other countries. All kinds of people have to work together to keep a hospital running smoothly both day and night. The book is illustrated throughout with photographs.
S, NF

65 HOW IT FEELS TO FIGHT FOR YOUR LIFE
Krementz, Jill
Victor Gollancz, 1990, 0 575 04770 4 Hb
For this collection of articles the author interviewed a number of children and young people who suffer from a chronic illness or disability, some of which are life-threatening. The children explain their feelings and discuss treatments, diets, exercises and schooling. The ages of those interviewed range from seven to sixteen, and their conditions vary from epilepsy to paraplegia.
S, NF

66 HOW TO LIVE WITH DIABETES
Dolger, Henry & Seeman, Bernard
Penguin, 1984, rev ed., 0 14 046501 4 Pb
A handbook on the diagnosis of the disease, its symptoms and treatment. There is discussion on methods of treatment, hereditary aspects of the condition and new developments in medication. The information given

is written clearly and concisely. Although originally published in America, it is updated regularly and adapted for the British market.
A, NF

67   I AM BLIND
Pettenuzzo, Brenda
Fairclough, Chris
Franklin Watts, 1988, 0 86313 698 2 Hb
Nigel was not born blind, but gradually lost his sight over a period of time. He is shown with his family and also at a residential school. Although Nigel learnt to read using print, he is also a braille reader. He swims, roller skates, and generally takes part in whatever is going on.
Lp, Up, NF

68   I AM DEAF
Pettenuzzo, Brenda
Murray, Maggie
Franklin Watts, 1987, 0 86313 571 4 Hb
Amina and her three brothers are all deaf. She is shown wearing a post-aural hearing aid and using a portable induction loop at school. The book explains how Amina and her brothers had their hearing loss diagnosed, in Amina's case at five years of age. Amina goes to a mainstream primary school and has no problems taking part in activities with her friends, including playing the recorder with a school group. Some facts about the ears and hearing are given at the end of the book.
Lp, Up, NF

69   I CAN SEE
Curry, Peter
Picture Lions, 1983, 0 00 662053 1 Pb
A celebration of sight for very young children which lists some of the things we see with our eyes. The illustrations are large, bright and colourful, and the text is clear.
I, Lp, Pic

70 I CAN'T ALWAYS HEAR YOU
Zelonky, Joy
Bejna, Barbara & Jensen, Shirlee
Blackwell Raintree, 1982, 0 86256 009 8 Hb
Kim is partially deaf and has just started mainstream school. She is the only child in school who wears a hearing aid and doesn't like to be different. Some of the children laugh when her speech doesn't sound right. The teacher explains about Kim's deafness and that she might have trouble with some sounds. However, Kim gets a very pleasant surprise when she discovers the headteacher also wears a hearing aid.
Lp, Up, F

71 I HAVE ASTHMA
Pettenuzzo, Brenda
Fairclough, Chris
Franklin Watts, 1989, 0 86313 745 8 Hb
Alexander is nine and has asthma. We follow him as he plays with his friends, goes to school, the cub scouts, and on holiday. Information is given on asthma, possible causes, medicines taken, but more importantly the book shows how normal his life is.
I, Lp, NF

72 I HAVE DIABETES
Althea
Dinosaur Pubs., 1992, 0 85122 809 7 Pb
A very simple introduction to diabetes.
Ps, I, NF

73 I HAVE DIABETES
Pettenuzzo, Brenda
Fairclough, Chris
Franklin Watts, 1987, 0 86313 561 7 Hb
Marcus has diabetes, but this does not stop him getting on with his life like any other ten-year-old boy. He describes how his parents suspected he might have diabetes, the tests that were done at the hospital. Marcus has to eat regular meals and snacks in between, and he has to work out the energy value of each food so that he has a balanced diet. Twice a day

he injects himself with insulin. He is also shown taking a blood sample and testing it for the sugar level.
Lp, Up, NF

74 I HAVE ECZEMA
Althea
Altham, Sarah
Dinosaur Publications, 1988, 0 85122 712 0 Pb
A girl explains that 'eczema is like being covered from head to toe with an itchy rash. It is not catching but it is very irritating'. She is allergic to some foods and certain types of fabrics such as wool, which makes her itch. Cotton clothing is the best. She swims and plays just like any other child, but has to take a little extra care by putting emollient on her skin after swimming.
I, Lp, Up, NF

75 I HAVE EPILEPSY
Althea
Dinosaur Pubs., 1991, 0 85122 818 6 Hb
A book which can be used with young children to explain epilepsy. It starts with a young child being diagnosed as epileptic and being given medicine to help control the fits. The child can do the same things as his friends, with the exception of riding a bike and climbing. This book will help to reassure a child.
I, Lp, NF

76 I HAVE EPILEPSY
Pettenuzzo, Brenda
Fairclough, Chris
Franklin Watts, 1989, 0 86313 8705 Hb
Salvatore Conte is eleven, and this photographic book follows him as he goes to school, plays, and takes part in ordinary activities. The only thing different about Salvatore is that he has epilepsy. He was diagnosed as epileptic at age nine after falling down while playing with some friends who could not wake him. An explanation of the different types of epilepsy is given and how fits can be triggered. In Salvatore's case very bright lights and flickering TV or VDU screens can induce a fit. He still

watches TV and plays with computers but takes extra care. Salvatore has to take pills every day to control the epilepsy.
Up, S, NF

77   IMRAN'S CLINIC
Teague, Kati
Magi Pubs., 1991, 1 85430 197 7 Pb, English
Magi Pubs., 1991, 1 84430 219 1 Hb, English
Magi Pubs., 1991, 1 85430 213 2 Hb, English/Gujarati
Magi Pubs., 1991, 1 85430 217 5, Hb, English/Urdu
Magi Pubs., 1991, 1 85430 214 0 Hb, English/Hindi
Magi Pubs., 1991, 1 85430 212 4 Hb, English/Greek
Magi Pubs., 1991, 1 85430 216 7 Hb, English/Turkish
Magi Pubs., 1991, 1 85430 215 9 Hb, English/Punjabi
Magi Pubs., 1991, 1 85430 210 8 Hb, English/Bengali
Magi Pubs., 1991, 1 85430 211 6 Hb, English/Chinese
Magi Pubs., 1991, 1 85430 218 3 Hb, English/Vietnamese
Imran and his mum take baby Jay to the clinic for a regular checkup and to have an inoculation. Imran is worried that the injection will hurt his brother, but the doctor reassures him it will only hurt for a moment. When Imran goes home, he and his friends play doctors and nurses.
Ps, I, Pic

78   IN STITCHES WITH MS WIZ
Blacker, Terence
Goffe, Toni
Piccadilly Press, 1989, 1 85340 044 0 Hb
Pan Books, 1990, 0 330 31222 7 Pb
Jack is rushed into hospital to have his appendix removed. One of the doctors turns out to be Ms Wiz who is a witch and whom Jack has met before. His hospital stay is made most enjoyable by the tricks that Ms Wiz plays on the doctors and nurses.
Lp, Up, F

79 INFECTIONS AND IMMUNISATION OF YOUR CHILD
Illingworth, Ronald S
Churchill Livingstone, 1981, 0 443 02238 0 Pb
The subject of immunisation attracts much controversy, with conflicting opinions and evidence making it difficult for parents to decide on vaccinations for childhood diseases. This slim volume gives equal weight to all opinions, allowing parents to come to a rational decision based on accurate information. In addition to childhood immunisation, vaccinations for travel abroad are also discussed, including the precautions necessary when travelling with children.
A, NF

80 INTO THE DARK
Wilde, Nicholas
Lions, 1989, 0 00 673517 7 Pb
Matthew is blind and dependent on his mother who is fearful of allowing him freedom. On holiday in Norfolk, Matthew meets Roly who introduces him to the marshes and the sea, to freedom of movement and a sense of exploration and independence. But Roly is a ghost; someone who can't be seen, even though he is very real to Matthew.
Up, S, F

81 IS DAD CRAZY?
Liddicut, Jan
McKay, Linda
Schizophrenia Australia, 1989, 1 875182 03 9 Hb
Schizophrenia is an illness which can be very frightening, not least to those most closely involved with the sufferer. A child is not able to rationalise the changed behaviour of adults, especially the changed character of a parent. By using a story technique, the author is able to help children understand by allowing the family to explain what is happening to their much-loved husband and father. The awful time before diagnosis, and the relief of discovering that their father is ill, are recorded in the children's thoughts and actions and their discussions with the doctor and their mother.
Up, A, NF

82 JASON BREAKS HIS ARM
Snell, Nigel
Hamish Hamilton, 1984, 0 241 11296 6 Hb
Jason falls from a rope swing and breaks his arm. His mother calls the ambulance and they go to the hospital. There his arm is X-rayed and a plaster put on, but he has to stay in overnight. When he gets back to school, he tells all his friends about his experiences and they all sign the plaster cast.
I, NF

83 JIMMY GOES TO THE DENTIST
Wade, Barry
Fairclough, Chris
Hamish Hamilton, 1984, 0 241 11300 8 Hb
A visit to the dentist to get a tooth filled turns out to be not as terrible an experience as Jimmy had envisaged. The dentist explains to Jimmy all the steps that she is taking to repair the tooth. When his treatment is finished she explains how he should look after his teeth so he won't get any more holes.
I, Lp, NF

84 JOHNNY GETS SOME GLASSES
Snell, Nigel
Hamish Hamilton, 1983, 0 241 89917 6 Hb
Hamish Hamilton, 1984, 0 241 11194 3 Pb
This series of books covers common experiences in childhood. In this title Johnny is taken to have his sight tested and as a result is given glasses to wear.
I, Lp, NF

85 KATE VISITS THE DOCTOR
Snell, Nigel
Hamish Hamilton, 1981, 0 241 10640 0 Hb
Hamish Hamilton, 1984, 0 241 11193 5 Pb
Kate wakes up one morning with an earache and her mother takes her to the doctor. The doctor examines Kate's chest, throat and ears, then checks her temperature with a thermometer, and writes out a prescription. They then go to the chemist and get the medicine.
Ps, I, NF

86 KATHY'S HATS
Krisher, Trudy
Westcott, Nadine Bernard
Albert Whitman, 1992, 0 8075 4116 8 Hb
Having loved hats all her young life, Kathy grows to hate them when her hair falls out following chemotherapy treatment for cancer. With her mother's help she thinks of a positive way to use her hats.
Lp, Up, Pic

87 KIM HAS ECZEMA
Pattison, Andrew
Barrett, Virginia
Hyland House, 1988, 0 947062 34 3 Hb
Kim doesn't want to go swimming because she is embarrassed by her eczema. Recently it has been very itchy and she has been scratching, so her arms and legs look all red and sore. The doctor gives her a checkup, and suggests a different cream. The doctor explains what eczema is and tells Kim that as she gets older the problem could disappear.
I, Lp, NF

88 THE KING'S TOOTHACHE
West, Colin
Dalton, Anne
Walker Books, 1987, 0 7445 0562 3 Hb
One day the King wakes up with toothache but no dentist can be found, so the baker and Town Crier are roped in to help. They only make matters worse. But when the sailor is asked to help the problem is solved. The story is told in rhyming four-line verses.
I, Lp, Pic

89 LINDA GOES TO HOSPITAL
Wade, Barry
Fairclough, Chris
A&C Black, 1981, 0 7136 2154 0 Hb
Linda's throat has been very sore and the doctor says that her tonsils are infected. She must go into hospital to have them removed. This photographic book shows all the stages from packing her bag, and being admitted, through having a checkup, being prepared for the operation

and having the operation, to recovery and aftercare before being sent home.
I, Lp, NF

90 THE LION WHO HAD ASTHMA
London, Jonathan
Westcott, Nadine Bernard
Albert Whitman, 1992, 0 8075 459 7 Hb
Like any other small boy, Sean has a vivid imagination. He likes to pretend to be an animal, and while being a lion suffers an asthma attack. To help the 'lion' breathe, Mum connects the nebuliser, and encourages Sean to be a jet pilot while wearing the oxygen mask through which the bronchodilating medicine is administered. As Sean breathes deeply through the machine, his wheezing is gradually controlled, until he can again be the 'lion in the jungle' and roar loudly.
I, Lp, Pic

91 LISTEN TO ME!
Mezei, Kathy
Voice, 1985, Pb
Amanda sometimes doesn't hear what people are saying and is frustrated when she can't pronounce some words clearly. She wears a hearing aid but doesn't like it because it makes her different from the other children. Her mother explains about her deafness and encourages her to use the hearing aid more so that she can hear better.
I, Lp, NF

92 LIVING WITH ALLERGIES
White, Dr T
Franklin Watts, 1990, 0 7496 0098 5 Hb
In simple language, and using both line drawings and photographs, this book explains some of the causes of allergies. The treatment of different allergies is explained and some of the side effects discussed. Both diet and medication are considered as treatment. There is a glossary of terms and also a brief listing of helpful organisations.
Up, S, A, NF

93 LIVING WITH ARTHRITIS
Shenkman, Dr John
Franklin Watts, 1990, 0 7496 0100 0 Hb
One of a series of titles dealing with disability, illness and handicap. Using good illustrations together with simple and accurate text, the author explains the condition known as arthritis. Various forms of treatment are discussed and illustrated, including surgery, physical therapy and alternative medicine such as acupuncture. Sufferers are shown going about their normal daily lives, and advice is given on avoiding injuries which could result in arthritis in later life.
Up, S, A, NF

94 LIVING WITH BLINDNESS
Parker, Steve
Franklin Watts, 1989, 0 7496 0043 8 Hb
One of a series which look at contemporary issues in health and disability. The text of this title discusses attitudes towards blindness, the diagnosis and treatment of sight difficulties, and advances in microelectronics which can help people with poor sight. The text is supported and extended through the use of photographs and diagrams.
Up, S, NF

95 LIVING WITH DEAFNESS
Taylor, Barbara
Franklin Watts, 1989 0 7496 0042 X Hb
An explanation of how the ears work which includes a clear cut-away diagram of the ear with all relevant parts labelled. The following chapters look at the different problems that can occur with the ear and how they can be treated. One chapter looks at deafness in detail, including sign language and lip reading. The final chapter discusses how to care for your ears e.g. avoiding excessive noise. This book also contains pictures of a grommet and shows how it is inserted into the eardrum.
Up, S, NF

96 LIVING WITH DIABETES
Taylor, Barbara
Franklin Watts, 1989, 0 7496 0044 6 Hb
A book aimed at the older child, with use of more scientific language to

explain diabetes. Different sections look at the various types of diabetes and the disorders that can result, the various kinds of treatment given, and how to live with diabetes.

Up, S, NF

97   LIVING WITH HEART DISEASE
Parker, Steve
Franklin Watts, 1989, 0 7496 0045 4 Hb
Using short well-illustrated paragraphs, this book outlines the various ways in which heart disease can affect people, from newborn babies to the elderly. There is discussion of medical intervention from bypass operations to major heart surgery, including valve replacement and heart transplant. There are general sections on healthy living, and caring for someone with a heart problem.

Up, S, A, NF

98   THE LONELY BASILISK
Lyons, Greg
Robinson, Colin
Hodder & Stoughton, 1989, 0 340 49715 7 Hb
Printed in large clear type and illustrated with line drawings, this is the story of a girl whose blindness helps her to understand the monster that lives in the cellar.

Lp, Up, Fic

99   MEDICINE
Aylett, John
Hodder & Stoughton, 1990, 0 340 49942 7 Hb
A look at how medicine and the treatment of disease in the UK has changed between 1901 and the present day. There are fourteen chapters dealing with such topics as government action, operations at home, vaccines, National Health Service, alternative medicine, and new problems such as AIDS.

Up, S, NF

100 MEDICINES AND DRUGS: BRITISH MEDICAL ASSOCIATION GUIDE
Henry, Dr John, (ed.)
Dorling Kindersley, 1991, 2nd ed., *0 86318 612 2* Hb
Dorling Kindersley, 1991, 2nd ed., *0 86318 679 3* Pb
A family reference book of commonly used medicines. It is efficiently indexed by generic and common drug names, and includes over 2,000 individual drugs. Each entry includes all alternative names for the drug, plus general comments and information for using the drug — the time it takes for any effect to be felt, possible adverse effects, and any special precautions needed. A system of visual codes allows the user to see quickly if the drug is suitable for use by children.
A, NF

101 MIFFY AND OTHERS IN HOSPITAL
Schlenther, Elizabeth
Haigh & Hochland, 1988, *1 869888 01 4* Pb
A brief paper on the need for, and the setting up of, book collections for children who are hospitalised. Areas covered include the selection and purchase of books, funding the collection and liaising with the hospital staff. One or two case studies are given, and the therapeutic value and use of books is mentioned. A very limited bibliography of books is included.
A, NF

102 MIFFY IN THE HOSPITAL
Bruna, Dick
Methuen, 1976, *0 416 57110 7* Hb
Miffy has a sore throat and the doctor tells her that she needs to go into hospital to have her tonsils removed. Only the most basic facts are given, and the whole tone is one of reassurance. This is for use with children under five years of age.
Ps, I, Pic

103 MIKE
Marshall, Margaret
Spiro, Lorraine
Bodley Head, 1983, *0 370 30934 0* Hb
Mike used to wet his bed a lot at night, but is slowly getting better. The

doctor explains some of the causes — being unhappy or worried, sleeping so deeply that you can't wake up in time to go to the lavatory. Mike tells the doctor he is afraid of the dark, so mum and dad give him a night light. A special pad with a buzzer is also put in the bed. The buzzer wakes Mike up if any moisture touches the pad.
I, Lp, NF

104 MISS DOSE THE DOCTOR'S DAUGHTER
Ahlberg, Allan
Jaques, Faith
Viking Kestrel, 1988, 0 670 81692 2 Hb
Puffin, 1988, 0 14 032346 5 Pb
Dora's parents are both doctors, and in this amusing tale Dora has to look after them and their patients when they both become ill. The patients think she is wonderful though they have never seen such a young doctor before. Eventually Dora catches the same illness her parents have and goes to bed, but mum and dad are now well enough to look after her.
I, Lp, F

105 MOG'S MUMPS
Nicoll, Helen
Pienkowski, Jan
Heinemann, 1977, 0 434 95640 6 Hb
Picture Puffin, 1981, 0 14 050357 9 Pb
Mog the cat has mumps. Meg and Owl look after him and they brew a wonderful medicine which cures Mog, but has some amusing side effects.
Ps, I, Pic

106 MUMMY GOES INTO HOSPITAL
Elliott, Evelyn
Cormack, Christopher
Hamish Hamilton, 1985, 0 241 11475 6 Hb
This is a useful book which shows a mother going into hospital. One of the children has already been in hospital so he knows that it is a nice place. Mum explains that she is going to have an operation to remove a small lump in her stomach. The children all help her pack her suitcase and then dad drives them to the hospital. The next morning mum has the

operation and they are able to visit her in the evening. She is on a drip and tells the children why and how it works. Dad is staying at home to look after the children while mum is in hospital and they all miss her. Eventually the day comes when they pack a suitcase with her going-home clothes.
I, Lp, NF

107 MY VISIT TO THE DENTIST
Bentley, Diana
Seheult, Paul
Wayland, 1989, 1 85210 716 2 Hb
A brief introduction to the work of a dentist, using photographs. These show the equipment he uses and the people who work with him, the receptionist, and the dental nurse. A glossary of key words is given at the back of the book.
I, Lp, NF

108 NICK HAS TONSILLITIS
Pattison, Andrew
Barrett, Virginia
Hyland House, 1988, 0 947062 31 9 Hb
Nick doesn't like having tonsillitis because it makes his throat so sore. He has to take a course of penicillin syrup. Being ill does have its rewards — he is allowed to eat lots of ice cream and jelly and stay away from school for a few days.
I, Lp, NF

109 NOW I UNDERSTAND
Lamore, Gregory S
Ensing-Keelean, Jan
Gaullaudet College Press, 1986, 0 930323 13 0 Pb
A new boy has joined the class and the teacher explains that he is deaf. Through simulation activities with the children the teacher shows them what it is like to be deaf. They cover their ears with their hands to try and understand how Jeff might hear sound, and learn how difficult it can be to lip-read. The children are shown some basic skills in communicating in sign language (in this case Amslan), how the ears work, and what a

hearing aid does. In the end the class has a better understanding of deafness.
Up, NF

110 NURSE
Cooper, Alison and Bentley, Diana
Fairclough, Chris
Wayland, 1990, 1 85210 849 5 Hb
Tony is a male charge nurse in the accident unit of a hospital. He has just come on duty and first of all he hears about the people who have been treated on the last shift. Alex has hurt her arm and has been brought in by mum. She has to sit in the waiting room until a doctor is free to see her. The doctor sends her for an X-ray, which confirms she has a broken wrist. Tony now has to put a plaster on her arm. Alex has also cut her leg, and after it is cleaned the nurse puts some stitches in. Finally Tony makes an appointment for Alex to come to the hospital clinic for a check up the following week.
I, Lp, Up, NF

111 THE NURSE
Stewart, Anne
Hamish Hamilton, 1984, 0 241 11162 5 Hb
A day in the life of a staff nurse in a Birmingham hospital. Work starts at 7.30 a.m. when she looks at the medical records of all the patients she will be looking after. She then gives out medicine from the drugs trolley, helps the doctor while he is doing his rounds, admits a new patient and prepares another patient for the operating theatre. Finally it is time to go home to her family.
I, Lp, NF

112 NURSE
Wood, Tim
Fairclough, Chris
Franklin Watts, 1988, 0 86313 713 X Hb
A photographic account of a nurse at work in a hospital: giving out medicine, helping the doctor, writing up records.
I, Lp, NF

113 ONE BEAR IN HOSPITAL
Bucknall, Caroline
Macmillan, 1990, 0 333 52643 0 Hb
While having a bicycle race with his friends, Teddy has an accident and is taken to hospital in an ambulance. The X-ray shows he has a broken leg, which is put into plaster. He has to stay in hospital for a few days and doesn't like the food, but he enjoys playing with the other children. When he is allowed to go home, it is in a wheel-chair which he will have to use for a while. All his friends think this is great.
I, Lp, Pic

114 ONE DAY AT A TIME: CHILDREN LIVING WITH LEUKAEMIA
Bergman, Thomas
Gareth Stevens, 1989, 0 83687 064 6 Hb
A black-and-white photographic book, originally published in Sweden, showing Hanna and Frederick in hospital having tests and receiving treatment for cancer. All aspects of the testing and treatment are shown in honest detail, including the pain that the children go through. A book that needs to be used with an adult.
Lp, Up, NF

115 THE OPTICIAN
Stewart, Anne
Fairclough, Chris
Hamish Hamilton, 1986, 0 241 11941 3 Hb
Elizabeth is taken to the optician to have her eyes checked. Using photographs, the author shows how the ophthalmic optician tests Elizabeth's sight, and then prescribes glasses. Also shown is a man being fitted with contact lenses and an elderly person being checked for glaucoma.
I, Lp, Up, NF

116 THE PHYSIOTHERAPIST
Stewart, Anne
Fairclough, Chris
Hamish Hamilton, 1989, 0 241 12574 X Hb
Jenny works in a large London hospital as a paediatric physiotherapist.

She is photographed as she goes through her normal daily routine working with patients who range from a new born baby to a child needing muscle-strengthening exercises. In each case the text explains the child's need for help and the type of assistance that is given through physiotherapy.
Up, S, NF

117 PERKINS THE CAT WHO WAS MORE THAN A FRIEND
Yeatman, Linda
Gon, Adriano
Piccadilly Press, 1987, 0 946826 83 8 Hb
Perkins is named after the brailling machine David is learning to use. Some blind people have a guide dog, but David has a cat as his best friend. Returning from a holiday, David discovers that the cat he left behind is not the cat he comes home to, but he has difficulty in making anyone believe him. With help, he discovers what happened to Perkins, and is overjoyed when she returns home.
Lp, Up, F

118 PETER GETS A HEARING AID
Snell, Nigel
Hamish Hamilton, 1979 0 241 89918 4 Hb
Hamish Hamilton, 1984 0 241 11190 0 Pb
Peter is finding it difficult to hear what people are saying, so his mother takes him to the hospital to have some tests. He is partially deaf and will need a hearing aid. Moulds of his ear are made so that the earpiece will fit properly. The day comes when he tries the hearing aid for the first time and can hear people and sounds a lot more clearly.
I, Lp, NF

119 POISON! BEWARE!
Skidmore, Steve
Cassell, 1990, 0 304 31774 8 Hb
Cassell, 1991, 0 304 32531 7 Pb
This is not about illness, but about the prevention of accidents due to ignorance. The poisons discussed range from chemicals found in the home to poisonous plants in the garden. The format is clear and simple

using pictures and text to enforce the message. Included are smoking and alcohol, plus environmental poisons.
Up, S, A, NF

120 PUTTING YOU IN THE PICTURE: AN INFORMATION PACK ABOUT EPILEPSY
National Society for Epilepsy, 1992, Video & Book
This package is designed to be used as a teaching or information aid. The book gives supplementary information which can be used in discussion after the video has been seen. An older epileptic might like to watch the video and then discuss it with family and friends, or it could be used in class groups or local community organisations to raise awareness. The cartoons by Rolf Harris illustrate each point made and graphically describe the text. The information given is general rather than specific, but it does include a section explaining what to do should a friend or relative have a seizure.
Up, S, A, NF

121 ROB HAS ECZEMA
Snell, Nigel
Hamish Hamilton, 1989, 0 241 12503 0 Hb
Rob has started to feel very itchy so mum takes him to the doctor. The doctor thinks he might have eczema and she sends him to the hospital for some tests. The tests prove positive, so Rob has to use special creams on his body, take tablets and also put oil in the water when he has a bath, to ease the itchiness. Gradually the redness and itchiness become better.
I, Lp, NF

122 SALLY ANN GOES TO THE HOSPITAL
Dicks, Terrance
Beek, Deborah van der
Piccadilly Press, 1988, 1 85340 035 1 Hb
Hippo Books, 1990, 0 590 76191 9 Pb
Jane has a bad asthma attack in school which necessitates her admission into the local hospital. However, she doesn't respond to the treatment given and is transferred to Great Ormond Street Hospital. Sally Ann, the classroom doll who can come to life, goes to keep Jane company and they are able to help another patient take an interest in life.
Lp, F

123 SALLY CAN'T SEE
Petersen, Palle
A&C Black, 1976, *0 7136 161 X* Hb
Sally attends a residential school for blind children, where she learns not only to read braille but also to swim, jump, run, and to go shopping by herself. The text explains the way Sally uses her senses and the photographs show a confident girl living her life to the full.
Up, NF

124 SARAH SEES THE SCHOOL DOCTOR
Snell, Nigel
Hamish Hamilton, 1989, *0 241 12502 2* Hb
Sarah is a little nervous when she has to go and see the school doctor for her annual checkup. But with mummy there as well she finds it is not scary, and she is able to tell her friends that the doctor is very nice.
I, NF

125 SAY CHEESE
Dinan, Carolyn
Faber & Faber, 1985, *0 571 13643 5* Hb
Bill is the only child in his class who still has all his first teeth. The class photograph is going to be taken at the end of the week and all the other children have gaps in their teeth. Bill is determined to keep his mouth closed and not smile unless he loses a tooth. Will his loose tooth fall out in time?
I, Lp, Pic

126 SCREENING FOR HEARING IMPAIRMENT IN YOUNG CHILDREN
McCormack, Barry
Chapman & Hall, 1991, *0 412 43800 3* Pb
In clearly written language this book outlines the methods used to screen children of varying ages for hearing loss. Photographs show the tests being carried out. There are also examples of audiograms explaining what they show and how to read them. The final chapter mentions new methods of screening not in use at the time of publication, some of which are now more common in the larger hospitals.
A, NF

127 SEEING IN SPECIAL WAYS
Bergman, Thomas
Gareth Stevens Children's Books, 1989, 0 83687 063 8 Hb
A photographic essay of interviews with, and photographs of, children who have visual handicaps ranging from near total blindness to partial sight. Each child answers a number of questions about themselves and their view of the world.
Up, S, NF

128 SIGHT
Jackman, Wayne
Fairclough, Chris
Wayland, 1989, 1 85210 731 6 Hb
A simple introduction to sight, including how eyes work, what we can do to protect them, and a few optical illusions. Illustrated with photographs and line drawings, this includes a glossary and index.
Lp, Up, NF

129 SPECCY FOUR-EYES
Lloyd, Carole
Kerins, Anthony
Julia MacRae Books, 1991, 1 85681 080 1 Hb
Anna wears glasses and is not only terrorised by Ellie but worried about the school trip to Bath. While walking around the Roman Baths something happens which helps Anna to gain confidence in herself and also to have the strength to cope with Ellie's particular brand of humour.
Up, F

130 A SPECIAL CHILD IN THE FAMILY: LIVING WITH YOUR SICK OR DISABLED CHILD
Kimpton, Diana
Sheldon Press, 1990, 0 85969 607 3 Pb
A book for parents which includes ideas for dealing with some of the problems faced by families where one child is chronically ill or suffering from a disabling condition. Dealing with the extended family and friends, learning what questions to ask medical staff and others involved with the child, facing the outside world, hospitalisation, schooling and beyond, plus terminal illness are also discussed.
A, NF

131 SPELLHORN
Doherty, Berlie
Hamish Hamilton, 1989, 0 241 12624 X Hb
Collins, 1990, 0 00 673500 2 Pb
The Wild Ones gallop down one night and take Laura away to help them find the lost unicorn who can lead them back to the Wilderness. In her own world Laura is blind, but in their world she is the only one who can see. The time warp allows Laura to use her skills and still return home before she is missed.
Up, S, F

132 SPOT'S HOSPITAL VISIT
Hill, Eric
Tempo Books, 1988, TBC 9530, (Book & Cassette)
Heinemann, 1987, 0 434 94272 3 Hb
Spot, Tom and Helen go to the hospital to visit their friend Steve, who has broken his leg, to cheer him up and take him presents. Spot is worried that Steve's plaster cast must hurt but Steve reassures him that it doesn't. Spot writes his name on the cast, as do Tom and Helen. As usual, Spot gets up to mischief.
Ps, I, Pic

133 SUGAR MOUSE
Branfield, John
Victor Gollancz, 1982, 0 575 01508 X Hb
Sarah is twelve and for the past three years has had diabetes. She especially dislikes the daily injections of insulin she has to give herself. However there are plus points to her life; she has a pony and is allowed to keep the stray dog she finds. It is only through a crisis that she realises she has to come to terms with the diabetes and her situation.
S, F

134 TEDDY BEARS AND THE COLD CURE
Gretz, Susanna
Sage, Alison
A&C Black, 1986, 0 7136 2832 4 Hb
Hippo Books, 1986, 0 590 70469 9 Pb
William catches a cold and has to stay in bed. At first he doesn't like this,

but soon realises that all he has to do is shout and his family will rush to make his favourite food, play his favourite games and be very nice to him. However, when it snows and the others make a sledge and go to try it out, William's cold instantly disappears.
Ps, I, Pic

135   TEETH FOR CHARLIE
Allen, Joy
Duchesne, Janet
Hamish Hamilton, 1976, 0 241 89421 2 Hb
Charlie hates going to the dentist, even throwing away the appointment card when it comes. However, when he loses two front teeth in a football match he cannot get to the dentist fast enough to have false teeth made so that the gap will disappear.
Lp, Up, F

136   'THEY NEVER WANT TO TELL YOU': CHILDREN TALK ABOUT CANCER
Bearison, David J
Harvard University Press, 1991, 0 674 88370 5 Hb
This is a very frank collection of interviews and discussions with children who suffer from cancer. The author is a developmental psychologist and psychotherapist who encourages the children to express their doubts and fears, their anger and compassion for themselves and their families and friends. Each child talks of both hope and despair through treatment and remission and watching friends die.
A, NF

137   THIS LITTLE BABY'S FIRST TOOTH
Breeze, Lynn
Orchard Books, 1992, 1 85213 370 8 Hb
A delightful board book about a baby's first tooth.
Ps, Pic

138   THOMAS HAS ASTHMA
Pattison, Andrew
Barrett, Virginia
Hyland House, 1988, 0 947062 33 5 Hb
Thomas has a cold which is making breathing difficult. Mum is worried and takes him to see the doctor. The doctor says that Thomas has had an asthma attack. He explains to Thomas what asthma is and how he will help Thomas with different medicines. In the surgery Thomas uses a nebuliser. When he goes back for a checkup the next day he is given an inhaler to use and asked to come back in a few weeks to see how the medicine is working.
I, Lp, NF

139   TOM VISITS THE DENTIST
Snell, Nigel
Hamish Hamilton, 1979, 0 241 89919 2 Hb
Hamish Hamilton, 1984, 0 241 11189 7 Pb
Tom doesn't like to smile because he has gaps in his teeth and the front ones stick out. All is cured when he goes to the dentist who fills the gaps up. In addition the dentist explains that he will fit a brace on Tom's teeth which will help to straighten them.
I, Lp, NF

140   TOO YOUNG TO DIE
McDaniel, Luriene
Bantam Books, 1991, 0 553 40367 2 Pb
Melissa is sixteen and has discovered she has leukaemia. With the help of her family and friends she comes to terms with the changes in her life and with the treatment, including the fact that it may not be successful and she may die. A companion volume to *Goodbye Doesn't Mean Forever*.
S, F

141   THE TOOTH BALL
Pearce, Philippa
Ganly, Helen
Andre Deutsch, 1987, 0 233 98062 8 Hb
Picture Puffin, 1989, 0 14 050823 6 Hb
When Tim's tooth comes out he wraps it in some gold foil, then some silver paper. Other children and adults give him different items to wrap around the increasingly larger ball. Through the fun of making this tooth ball, Tim makes new friends.
I, Lp, Pic

142   THE TROUBLE WITH JOSH
Nystrom, Carolyn
Rees, Gary
Lion Pubs., 1989, 0 7459 1313 X Hb
Josh finds it difficult to sit still for longer than a few minutes. He also finds it hard to learn as his concentration span is very short. He takes medication to allow him to relax, but he still needs constant supervision. The author explains that hyperactivity is a condition which places severe strain on other family members as it is often misunderstood and regarded as bad behaviour. Like Josh, many of the children who suffer are quite bright in some academic subjects, but they find it hard to see the consequences of their actions until after the event.
Lp, NF

143   TWO WEEKS WITH THE QUEEN
Gleitzman, Morris
Pan Books, 1990, 0 330 31376 2 Hb
Colin and his family live in Australia. When his brother is diagnosed as having cancer, Colin is sent to stay with an aunt and uncle in London. Colin decides that the only way to help Luke is to go to the Queen. By befriending Ted whose friend is dying with AIDS, Colin comes to terms with the fact that Luke may also die.
Up, F

144 THE VIEW BEYOND MY FATHER
Allan, Mabel Esther
Firecrest, 1987, 0 85997 695 5 Hb
A blind girl, living under the restrictive influence of a domineering parent, battles to free herself. In her middle teens she is given the opportunity to continue that freedom through an operation to partially restore her sight. Set some time between the wars, this book explores the social acceptability of a child with a handicap and the way in which society in those days encouraged these children to be hidden.
S, F

145 VISIT TO THE HOSPITAL
Devane-Caveney, Clare
Byrnes, Lynne
World International, 1991, 0 7498 0116 6 Hb
Emily and her family have been to hospital for many different reasons — broken leg, having a baby, getting eyes tested, allergy checks, physiotherapy treatment. As Emily says, hospitals are good places which make people better.
I, Lp, NF

146 WAITING FOR BABY JOE
Collins, Pat Lowry
Dun, Jaon Whinham
Albert Whitman, 1990, 0 8075 8625 0 Hb
Missy waits anxiously for her premature baby brother to come home. While she waits she endures the mood changes of both parents and their preoccupation with Joe's fragile hold on life. Even when Joe does come home he has to be carefully watched by his parents and a monitoring machine. Not until he smiles and has his own striped T-shirt does Missy feel he is old enough to have a big sister.
Lp, Up, A, NF

147 WATCH OUT RONALD MORGAN
Giff, Patricia Reilly
Natti, Susanna
Viking Kestrel, 1985, 0 670 80433 9 Hb
Always in trouble for bumping, knocking things and being awkward,

Ronald Morgan's life changes for the better when he gets his first pair of glasses. Things don't improve miraculously, but he does begin to learn to read, and become more reliable when playing ball games.
I, Lp, F

148   WHAT DIFFERENCE DOES IT MAKE, DANNY?
Young, Helen
Blake, Quentin
Andre Deutsch, 1980, 0 233 97248 X Hb
Danny is an ordinary boy who likes sport and gets up to mischief. He has epilepsy but this doesn't bother him. A new teacher who doesn't understand epilepsy, arrives at school and it is up to Danny to help the teacher overcome his worries.
Up, F

149   WHAT HAPPENS WHEN YOU CATCH A COLD
Richardson, Joy
MacLean, Colin & Moira
Evans Bros., 1992, 0 2337 60199 0 Hb
A simple explanation of what a cold is, how the germs breed, what the viruses are and how colds are spread.
I, Lp, NF

150   WHAT'S UP, MATE?
Bales, Helen
Hodder & Stoughton, 1987, 0 340 35983 8 Hb
This book was written by a mother whose son, Anthony, died of cancer. Because she found it difficult to find information to explain cancer to her son, she decided to write this book. The story does not include Anthony's death, but ends with him in remission.
I, Lp, Up, NF

151   THE WITCH'S DAUGHTER
Bawden, Nina
Gollancz, 1966, 0 575 00177 1 Hb
Heinemann Educ., 1972, 0 435 12167 7 Hb
Puffin Books, 1969, 0 14 030407 X Pb
A novel set on a Scottish island in which the blind daughter of a witch

uses her second sight and her senses of touch and hearing to help solve a mystery. Ephemeral as a book about sight loss, but a good positive image of a blind child.
Up, S, F

152   WORKING IN A HOSPITAL
Storr, S D
Humphrey, Tim
Wayland, 1982, 0 85340 926 9 Hb
Many different people work in a hospital to ensure that it runs smoothly. In this book twelve different jobs are discussed. As well as a doctor and a nurse, the text mentions a cook, a scientific officer, a pharmacist, a dietician, a porter, an engineer, a radiographer, and an administrative assistant. Their jobs are explained, and also the training and qualifications that are required.
Up, S, NF

KEYWORD INDEX

To simplify the use of this handbook all entries are arranged alphabetically by title. This index allows the user to find a specific topic and go direct to the numbered entries given.

ACCIDENTS	1, 82, 113
AIDS see HIV: AIDS	
ALLERGIES	6, 29, 92
AMBULANCE	7, 8, 9, 82
ARTHRITIS	93
ASTHMA	5, 13, 26, 31, 61, 71, 90, 122, 138
BED WETTING	60, 103
BROKEN BONES	82, 113, 132
CANCER	2, 24, 53, 86, 114, 136, 140, 143, 150
CHICKENPOX	43
CHILDCARE	24, 25, 29, 34, 39, 42, 79, 100, 101, 119, 126, 130
CHRONIC ILLNESS	42, 65
COLDS	134, 149
DENTIST	17, 32, 48, 49, 83, 107, 139
DIABETES	33, 34, 40, 66, 72, 73, 96, 133, 148
DOCTOR	14, 18, 22, 23, 36, 41, 50, 51, 77, 85, 104, 124
DRUGS	100
EPILEPSY	38, 75, 76, 120
GERMS	45, 55, 149
GLASSES	15, 21, 30, 46, 84, 115, 129, 147
HAEMOPHILIA	25
HEALTH	35, 44, 55, 56, 119
HEARING	27, 28, 45, 52, 58, 59, 68, 70, 85, 91, 95, 109, 118, 126
HEARING AID	19, 68, 70, 91, 109, 118
HEARING DOG	20
HEART DISEASE	97
HICCUPS	62
HIV: AIDS	3, 4, 143
HOSPITAL	1, 16, 47, 52, 63, 64, 78, 82, 89, 101, 102, 106, 113, 122, 132, 143, 145, 146, 152
HYPERACTIVITY	6, 142
INFECTION	14, 27, 44, 50, 55, 79, 85, 89

INOCULATIONS	50, 51, 77, 79, 99
LEUKAEMIA see CANCER	
MEASLES	54
MEDICINE	100
MEDICINE — HISTORY	99
MUMPS	105
NURSE	110, 111, 112
OBESITY	37
OPTICIAN	15, 46, 84, 115
PHYSIOTHERAPIST	116
POISONS	119
PREMATURE BIRTH	146
SCHIZOPHRENIA	81
SIGHT	15, 21, 57, 67, 69, 80, 94, 98, 115, 117, 123, 127, 128, 129, 131, 144, 147, 151
SKIN DISORDERS	29, 74, 87, 121
SPEECH PROBLEMS	10, 28, 121
SPEECH THERAPIST	10
TEETH	11, 12, 88, 125, 135, 137, 141
TONSILS	89, 102, 108
TONSILLITIS	19
TOOTHACHE	26, 29
TOOTH LOSS	22, 23, 32, 33, 35

AUTHOR INDEX

The numbers refer to the individual entry numbers and not pages.

AHLBERG, Allan   104
ALLAN, Mabel Esther   144
ALLEN, Joy   135
ALTHEA   47, 72, 74, 75
AYLETT, John   99
AZARNOFF, Pat   56
BALES, Helen   150
BAWDEN, Nina   151
BEARISON, David J   136
BENTLEY, Diana   7, 107, 110
BERGER, Melvin   44
BERGMAN, Thomas   114, 127
BLACKER, Terrance   78
BRANFIELD, John   133
BREEZE, Lynn   137
BROWN, Laurie Krasny   35
BROWN, Marc   12, 35
BRUNA, Dick   25, 102
BUCKNALL, Caroline   113
CARLETON, Don   24
CIVARDI, Anne   48, 50, 52
COLHERNE, John   63
COLLINS, Pat Lowry   146
COOPER, Alison and BENTLEY, Diana   7, 110
CUNLIFFE, John   16
CURRY, Peter   69
CURTIS, Sarah   42
DEVANE-CAVENEY, Clare   145
DICKS, Terrance   122
DINAN, Carolyn   15, 125
DOHERTY, Berlie   131
DOLGER, Henry and SEEMAN, Bernard   66
ELLIOTT, Evelyn   106
FARQUHAR, J W   33, 34

FINE, Judy   2
GIFF, Patricia Reilly   147
GIRARD, Linda Walvoord   4
GLEITZMAN, Morris   143
GOLDMAN, Dara   62
GRETZ, Susanna   134
GRUNSELL, Angela   14
HAWKES, Nigel   3
HENRY, Dr John   100
HILL, Eric   132
HOBAN, Lillian   11
JACKMAN, Wayne   57, 58, 128
ILLINGWORTH, Ronald   79
KELLER, Holly   30
KIMPTON, Diana   130
KRAILING, Tessa   1
KREMENTZ, Jill   65
KRISHER, Trudy   86
LAIDLAW, John   39
LAIDLAW, Mary V   39
LAMORE, Gregory S   109
LEIGH, Dr Irene and WOJNAROWSKA, Dr Fenella   29
LIDDICUT, Jan   81
LIESHOUT, Ted Van   31
LITCHFIELD, Ada B   19, 21
LLOYD, Carole   129
LONDON, Jonathan   90
LYONS, Greg   98
McCORMACK, Barry   126
McDANIEL, Lurlene   53, 140
MARSHALL, Margaret   103
MAYNE, William   45
MEADOW, Roy   60
MEZEI, Kathy   91
MILNER, A D   13

NATIONAL SOCIETY FOR
  EPILEPSY   120
NICOLL, Helen   105
NYSTROM, Carolyn   142
OSTROW, William and Ostrow,
  Vivian   5
OXENBURY, Helen   22
PARKER, Steve   94, 97
PATTISON, Andrew   27, 36, 87, 108,
  138
PEARCE, Philippa   141
PEPPER, Susan   41
PETERSEN, Palle   123
PETTENUZO, Brenda   67, 68, 71, 73,
  76
PETTY, Kate   49, 51
PHILIPS, Barbara   37
PIRNER, Connie White   40
PLUCKROSE, Henry   59
POWLING, Chris   54
RAPP, Doris J   6
RICHARDSON, Joy   149
ROGAN, Peter   38
SCHLENTHER, Elizabeth   101
SEEMAN, Bernard   66

SHENKMAN, Dr John   93
SKIDMORE, Steve   119
SMITH, Katherine A   23
SMITH, Lane   46
SNELL, Nigel   10, 43, 82, 84, 85, 118,
  121, 124, 139
STEWART, Anne   9, 111, 115, 116
STORR, S D   152
SUTHERLAND, Susan   61
TAYLOR, Barbara   95, 96
TEAGUE, Kati   77
URE, Jean   28
VAUGHAN, Jenny   64
WADE, Barry   83, 89
WARD, Brian R   55
WEST, Annie   17, 18
WEST, Colin   88
WHITE, Dr T   92
WILDE, Nicholas   80
WOJNAROWSKA, Dr Fenella   see
  Leigh
WOOD, Tim   8, 32, 112
YEATMAN, Linda   20, 26, 117
YOUNG, Helen   148
ZELONKY, Joy   70

ORGANISATIONS AND THEIR ADDRESSES

These organisations offer help and advice to those caring for children. Most organisations have printed leaflets available. When writing for information, it is best to enclose a large stamped self-addressed envelope.

ACT
Institute of Child Health, Royal Hospital for Sick Children, St Michael's Hill, Bristol BS2 8BJ. Tel: 0272 221556

Help for families whose children have life-threatening and terminal illnesses.

ACTION AGAINST ALLERGY
24-26 High Street, Hampton Hill, Middlesex TW12 1PD

ACTION FOR SICK CHILDREN, (NAWCH)
Argyle House, 29-31 Euston Road, London NW1 2SD. Tel: 071 833 2041

ACTION FOR SICK CHILDREN — NORTHERN IRELAND
Branch is dormant at present. Contact London address for help.

ACTION FOR SICK CHILDREN — REPUBLIC OF IRELAND, (NAWCH)
Brookwood, Tuber, Lucan, Co. Dublin, Ireland. Tel: 0001 628 1157

ACTION FOR SICK CHILDREN — SCOTLAND
15 Smith's Place, Edinburgh EH6 8NT. Tel: 031 553 6553

All these organisations work for the welfare of children in hospital. Information sheets are available and designed to be used either by children alone, or by parents and professionals.

BLISS
17-21 Emerald Street, London WC1N 3QL. Tel: 071 831 9393

Support group for parents who have new-born babies needing intensive care.

BRITISH DIABETIC ASSOCIATION
10 Queen Anne Street, London W1M 0BD. Tel: 071 323 1531

BRITISH HEART FOUNDATION
14 Fitzharding Street, London W1H 4DH. Tel: 071 935 0185

CANCER AND LEUKAEMIA IN CHILDHOOD TRUST (CLIC)
CLIC House, 11-12 Freemantle Square, Cotham, Bristol BS6 5TL. Tel: 0272 244333
Support, information and advice for children with cancer and their families.

CANCER RELIEF MACMILLAN FUND
Anchor House, 15-19 Britten Street, London SW3 3TZ. Tel: 071 351 7811
Gives advice and information on home and hospice care.

COLLEGE OF SPEECH AND LANGUAGE THERAPISTS
7 Bath Place, Rivington Street, London EC2A 3DR. Tel: 071 613 3855

CRUSE
Cruse House, 126 Sheen Road, Richmond, Surrey TW9 1UR. Tel: 081 940 4818
Provides support and help for all bereaved persons, especially siblings.

DEPARTMENT OF SOCIAL SECURITY
Leaflets Unit, PO Box 21, Honeypot Lane, Stanmore, Middlesex HA7 8PS
Provides various guides.

DIABETES FOUNDATION
177A Tenison Road, London SE25 5NF. Tel: 081 656 5467

ENURESIS RESOURCE and INFORMATION CENTRE (ERIC)
65 St Michael's Hill, Bristol BS2 8DZ. Tel: 0272 264 920
Provides an information service to parents and professionals on bed-wetting. Produces various leaflets and will provide addresses of specialist advisors.

EPILEPSY ASSOCIATION — BRITISH
Anstey House, 40 Hanover Square, Leeds LS3 1BE. Tel: 0532 439393

EPILEPSY ASSOCIATION — NORTHERN IRELAND
Old Post-Graduate Medical Centre, City Hospital, Lisburn Road, Belfast BT9 7AF. Tel: 0232 248214

EPILEPSY ASSOCIATION — REPUBLIC OF IRELAND
249 Crumlin Road, Dublin 12. Tel: 0001 557500

EPILEPSY ASSOCIATION — SCOTLAND
48 Govan Road, Glasgow GS1 1JL. Tel: 041 427 4911

All branches of this organisation provide support, information, publications and assessment through regional offices and local support groups.

EPILEPSY FEDERATION
71 Stanley Road, Croydon, Surrey CR0 3QF. Tel: 081 665 1255
Information, support and assistance with setting up local groups.

EPILEPSY — NATIONAL SOCIETY FOR
Chalfont St Peter, Gerrards Cross, Buckinghamshire SL9 0RJ. Tel: 0494 873991
Will give advice on assessment, rehabilitation and care.

GENERAL DENTAL COUNCIL
37, Wimpole Street, London W1M 8DQ. Tel: 071 486 2171
Produce a catalogue on material about the dental world. Items suitable for use by children.

HAEMOPHILIA SOCIETY
123 Westminster Bridge Road, London SE1 7HR. Tel: 071 928 2020
Publishes a newsletter, and will provide information, literature, and support.

HEALTH SEARCH SCOTLAND
Health Education Board for Scotland, Woodburn House, Canaan Lane, Edinburgh EH10 4SG
Provides information via a computer database on self-help and voluntary groups throughout Scotland which work in the field of health. Also has a collection of information leaflets, booklets and a small resource centre housing books and journals aimed at the lay reader.

HOSPITAL PLAY STAFF SCOTLAND
c/o 15 Smith's Place, Edinburgh EH6 8NT. Tel: 031 553 2189

HYPERACTIVE CHILDREN'S SUPPORT GROUP (HCSG)
71 Whyke Lane, Chichester, West Sussex PO19 2LD. Tel: 0903 725182
A parental support group with branches in many areas of the country. Provides information including a handbook.

LEUKAEMIA CARE SOCIETY
14 Kingfisher Court, Venny Bridge, Pinhoe, Exeter, Devon EX4 8JN. Tel: 0392 64848

LOOK
National Federation of Families with Visually Impaired Children, Queen Alexandra College, 49 Court Oak Road, Birmingham B17 9TG. Tel: 021 428244

NATIONAL ASSOCIATION FOR HOSPITAL PLAY STAFF
Thomas Coram Foundation for Children, 40 Brunswick Square, London WC1. Tel: 071 278 2824

NATIONAL ASTHMA CAMPAIGN
Providence House, Providence Place, London N1 0PT. Tel: 071 226 2260

Works with both children and adults. Children can join the Junior Asthma Club aimed at 6-11 year olds, and receive regular copies of the magazine *A for Asthma*. The NAC provides literature and has local groups around the country.

NATIONAL DEAF CHILDREN'S SOCIETY (NDCS)
Family Services Centre, Carlton House, 24 Wakefield Road, Rothwell Haigh, Leeds LS26 0SF. Tel: 0532 823458 (voice or text)

Offers advice on all aspects of deaf children's education and welfare, including personal help with educational reviews and appeals. There is also an information service and library.

NATIONAL ECZEMA SOCIETY
4 Tavistock Place, London WC1H 9RA. Tel: 071 388 4097

Information, advice and publications.

NATIONAL SOCIETY FOR RESEARCH INTO ALLERGY
26 Welling Road, Hinckley, Leicestershire LE10 1JE

PARTIALLY SIGHTED SOCIETY
Queens Road, Doncaster, S. Yorkshire DN1 2NX. Tel: 0302 323132

PLAY IN SCOTTISH HOSPITALS
15 Smith's Place, Edinburgh EH6 8NT. Tel: 031 553 2189

Promotes organised therapeutic and diversionary play in hospitals, health centres and clinics in Scotland. Offers information, advice and training for hospital staff, parents and playworkers.

PLAY MATTERS
National Toy Libraries Association, 68 Churchway, London NW1 1LT. Tel: 071 387 9592

ROYAL NATIONAL INSTITUTE FOR THE BLIND
224 Great Portland Street, London W1N 6AA. Tel: 071 388 1266

ROYAL NATIONAL INSTITUTE FOR THE DEAF
105 Gower Street, London WC1E 6AH. Tel: 071 387 8033

ROYAL SOCIETY FOR MENTALLY HANDICAPPED CHILDREN AND ADULTS, (MENCAP)
117-123 Golden Lane, London EC1 0RF. Tel: 071 253 9433

TERENCE HIGGINS TRUST
52-54 Grays Inn Road, London WC1X 8JU. Tel: 071 831 0330

For all information on caring for people with AIDS.

VISION AID
22A Chorley New Road, Bolton, Lancashire BL1 4AP. Tel: 0204 31882.
A support group for parents who have a child who is partially sighted or blind.

VOCAL (Voluntary Organisations, Communication & Language)
336 Brixton Road, London SW9 7AA. Tel: 071 274 4029
An umbrella organisation for several charities and groups working in the field of speech and communication problems. Enquirers are referred to an appropriate source of help.

Tixylix Paediatric Medicines produce a booklet called 'Making it Better', a guide to caring for your sick child. Available from Tixylix, Intercare Products Ltd, Fishponds Road, Wokingham, Berks.